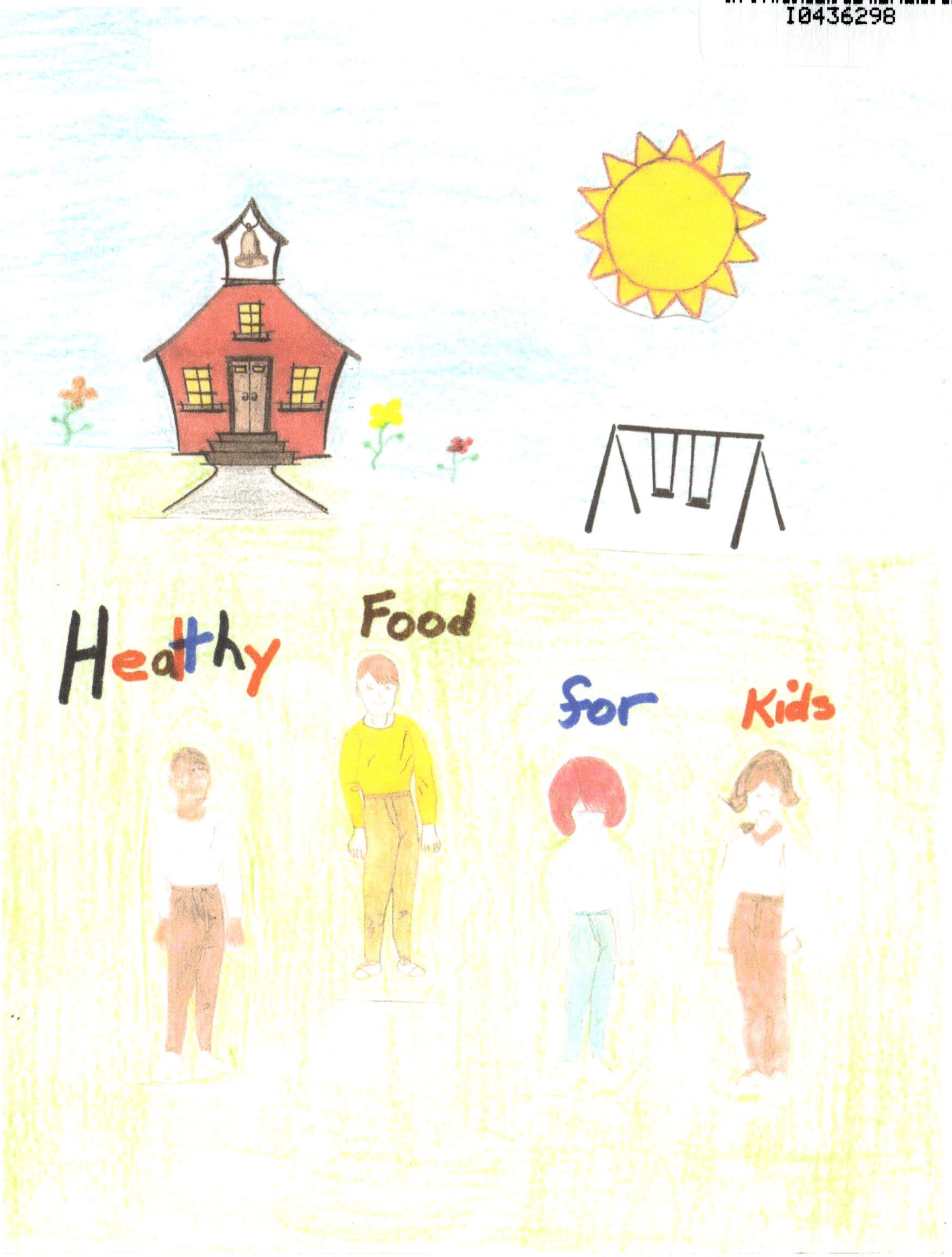

Healthy Food for Kids

Once there were two kids who had problems trying to lose weight.

Every day, the two kids got laughed at by all the other kids except two,

Mickey and Sandy.

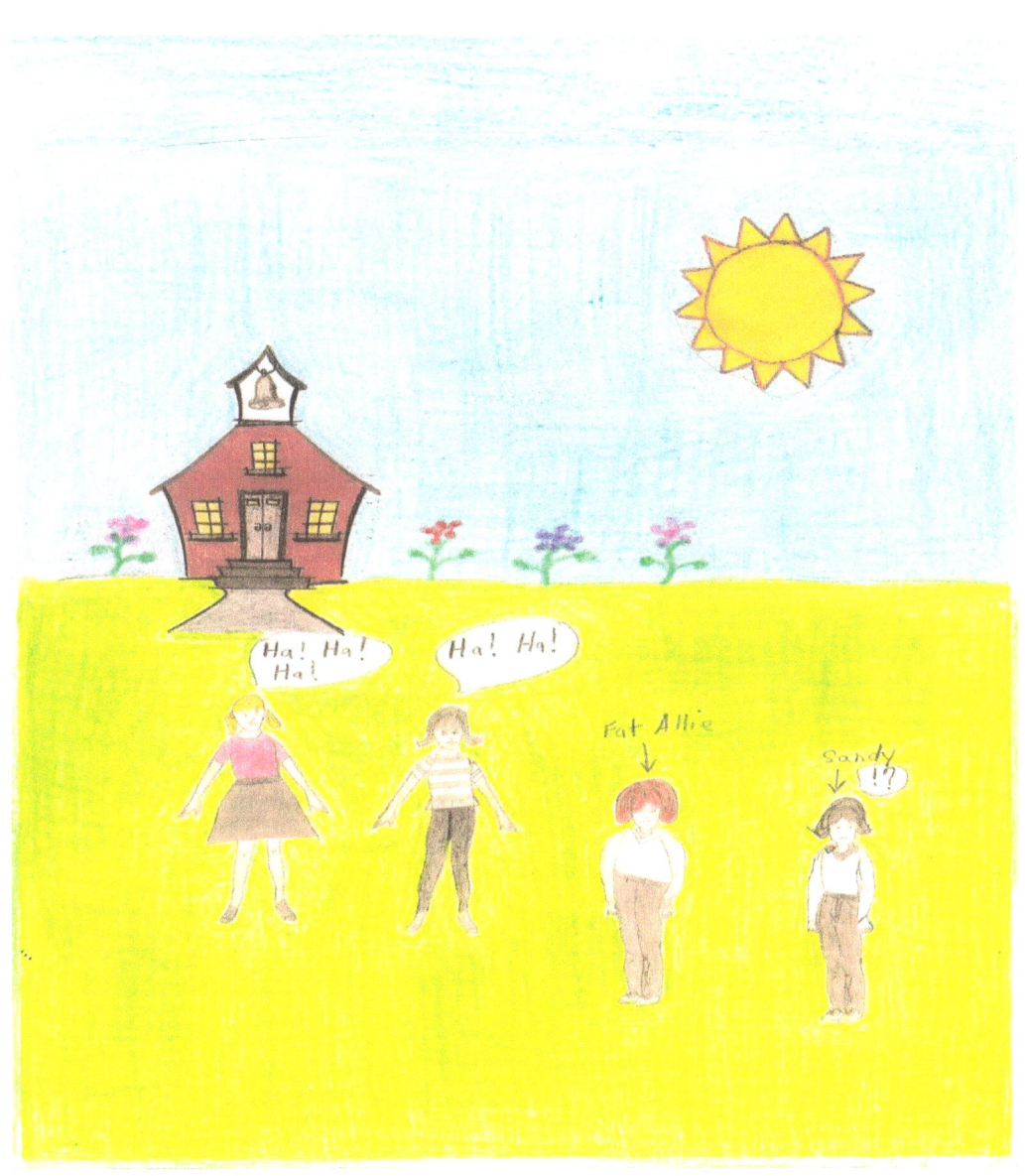

The kids in school had called, Tom, Tubby, and Allie, and the girl was called Fat Allie.

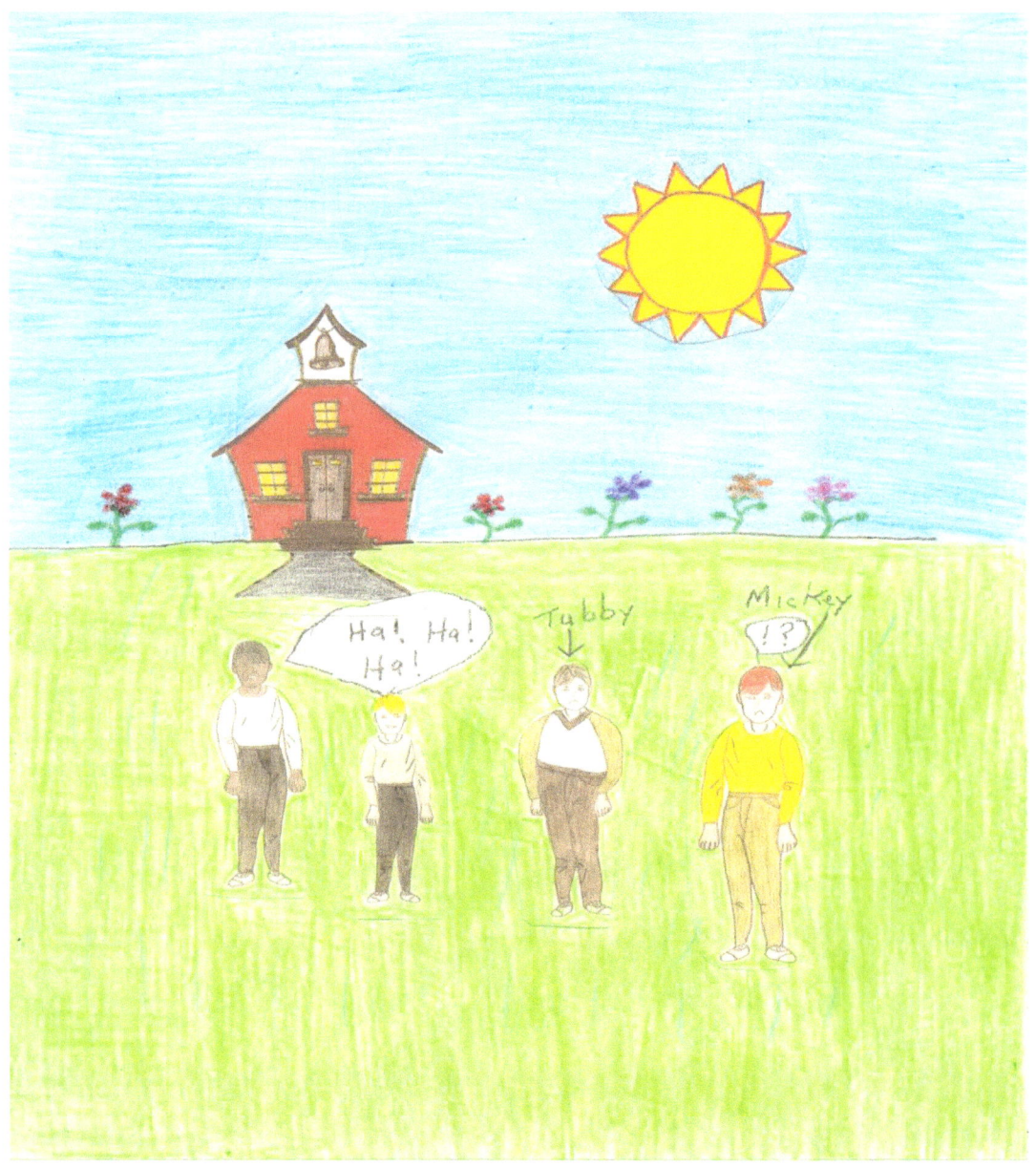

Sandy felt so bad, that she decided to spend time with Fat Allie by inviting her for lunch.

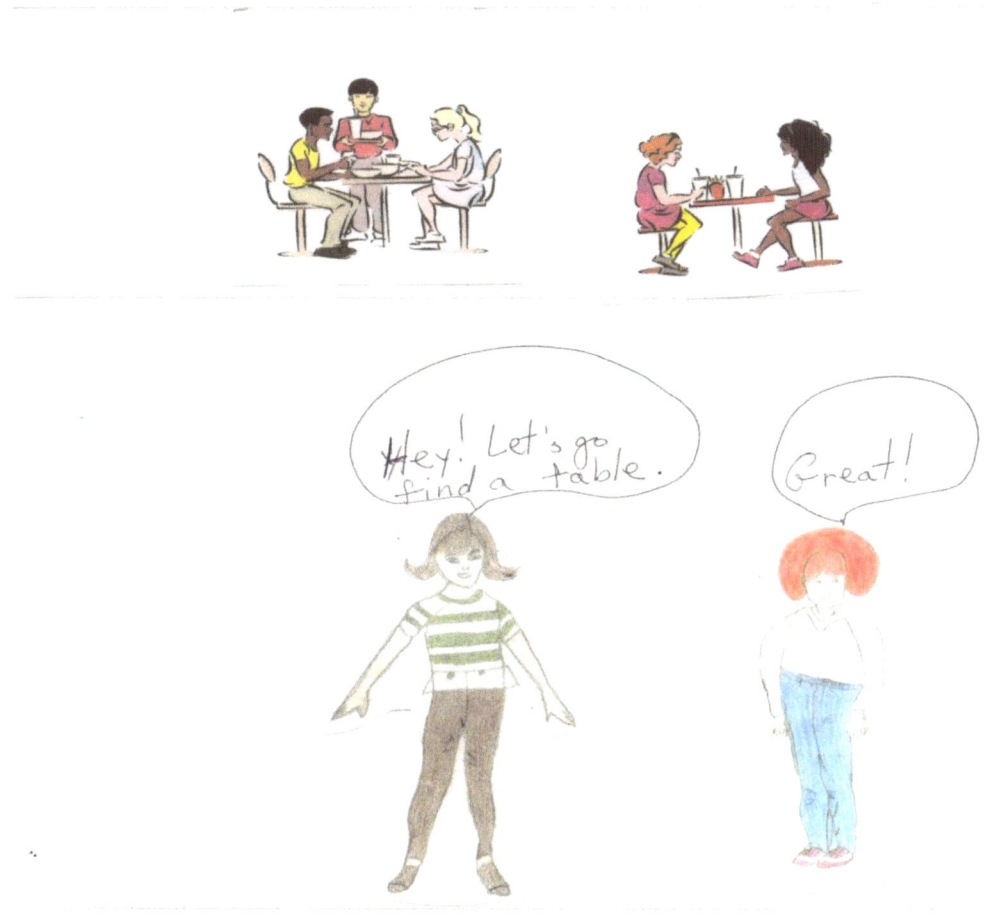

As for Tubby, Mickey did the same thing as Sandy.

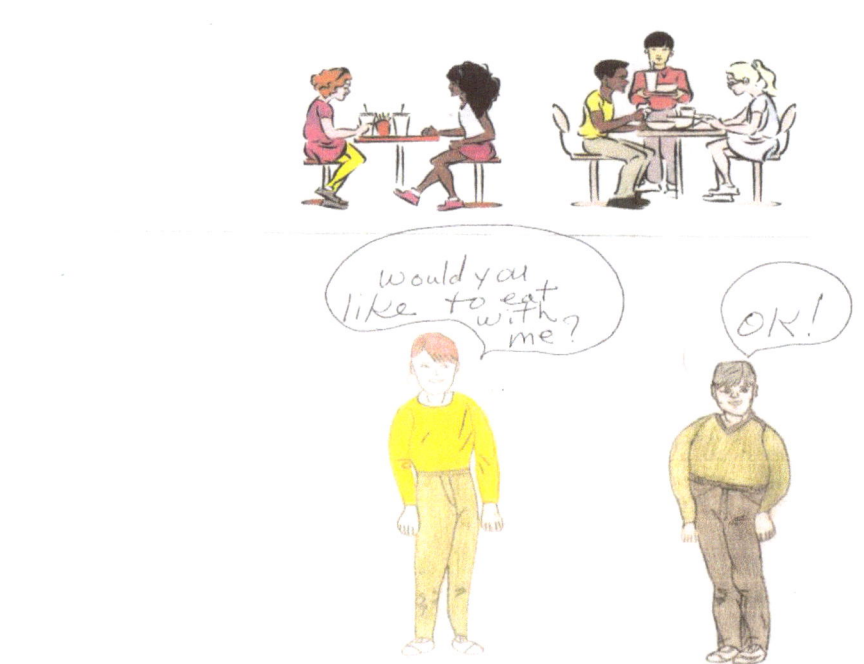

Sandy invited Fat Allie to play with her in the playground.

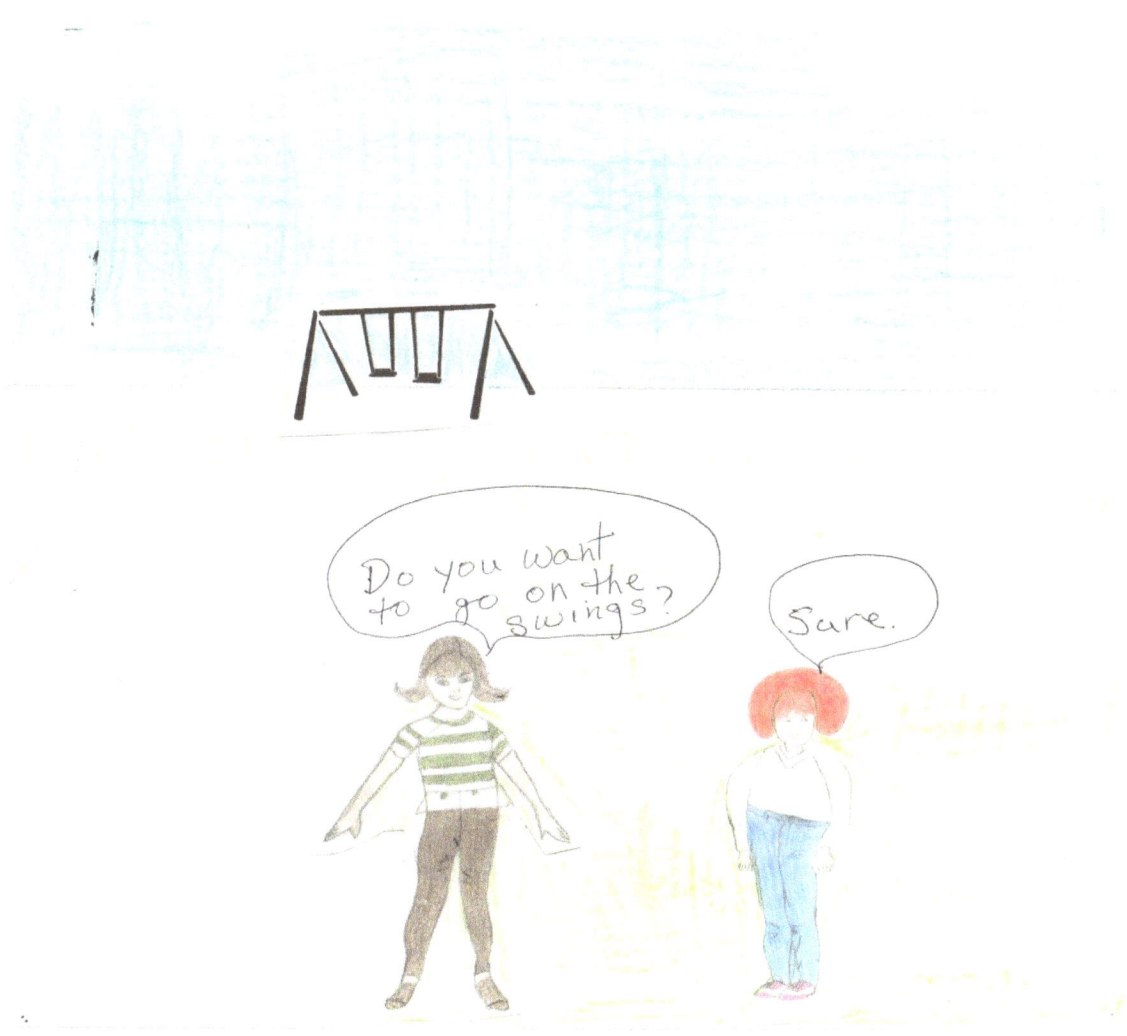

One day, Sandy invited Fat Allie to come to her house to play.

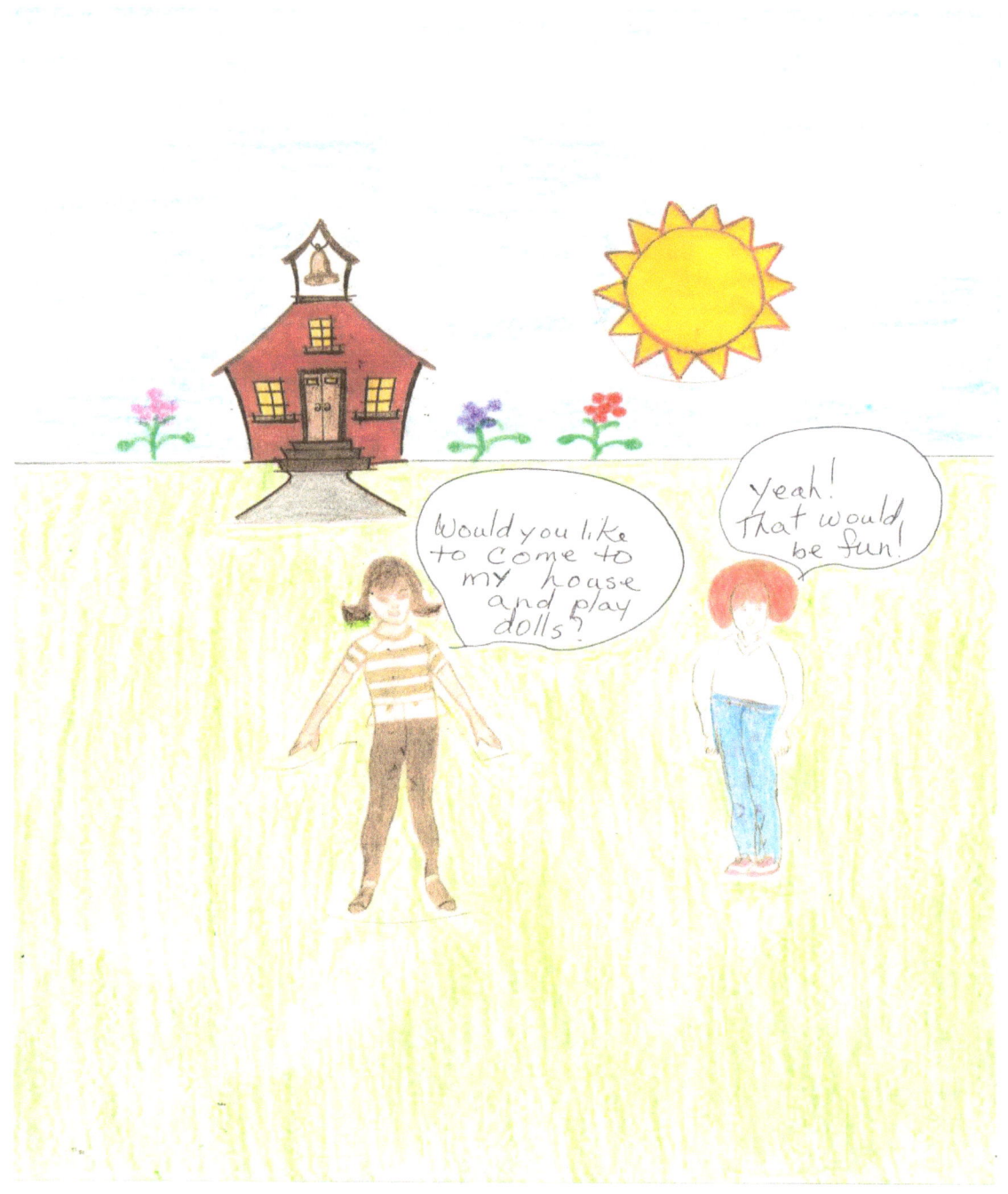

All the other girls told Sandy not to bother with Fat Allie.

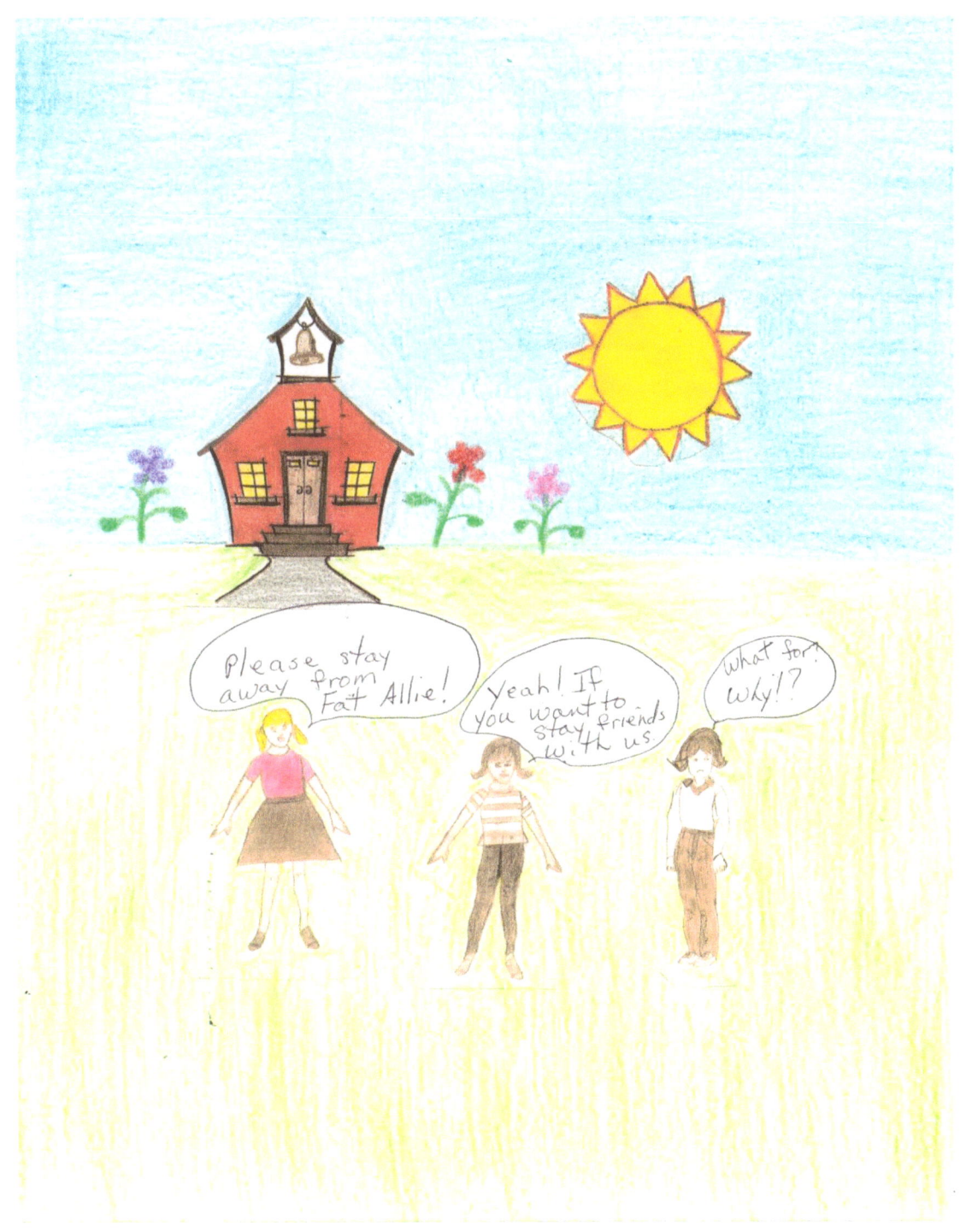

As for Mickey, he invited Tubby to play with him in the playground.

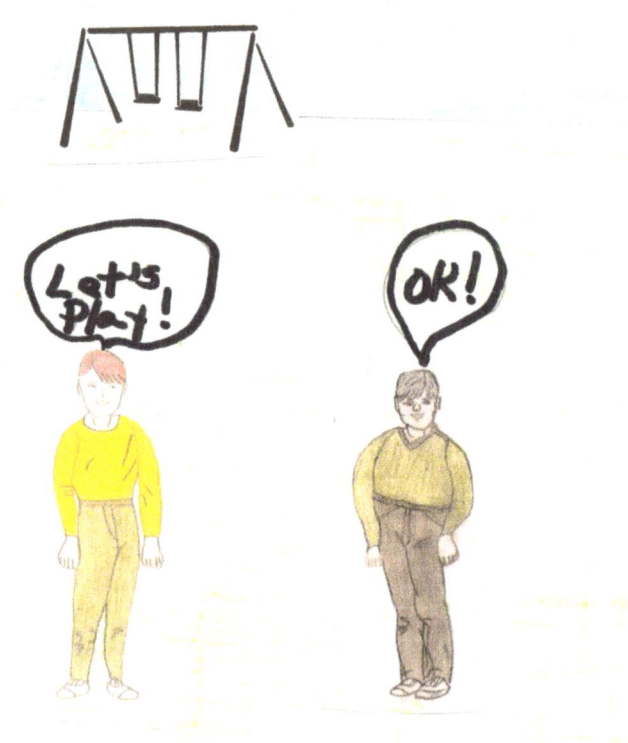

All of Mickey friends told him to stay away from Tubby.

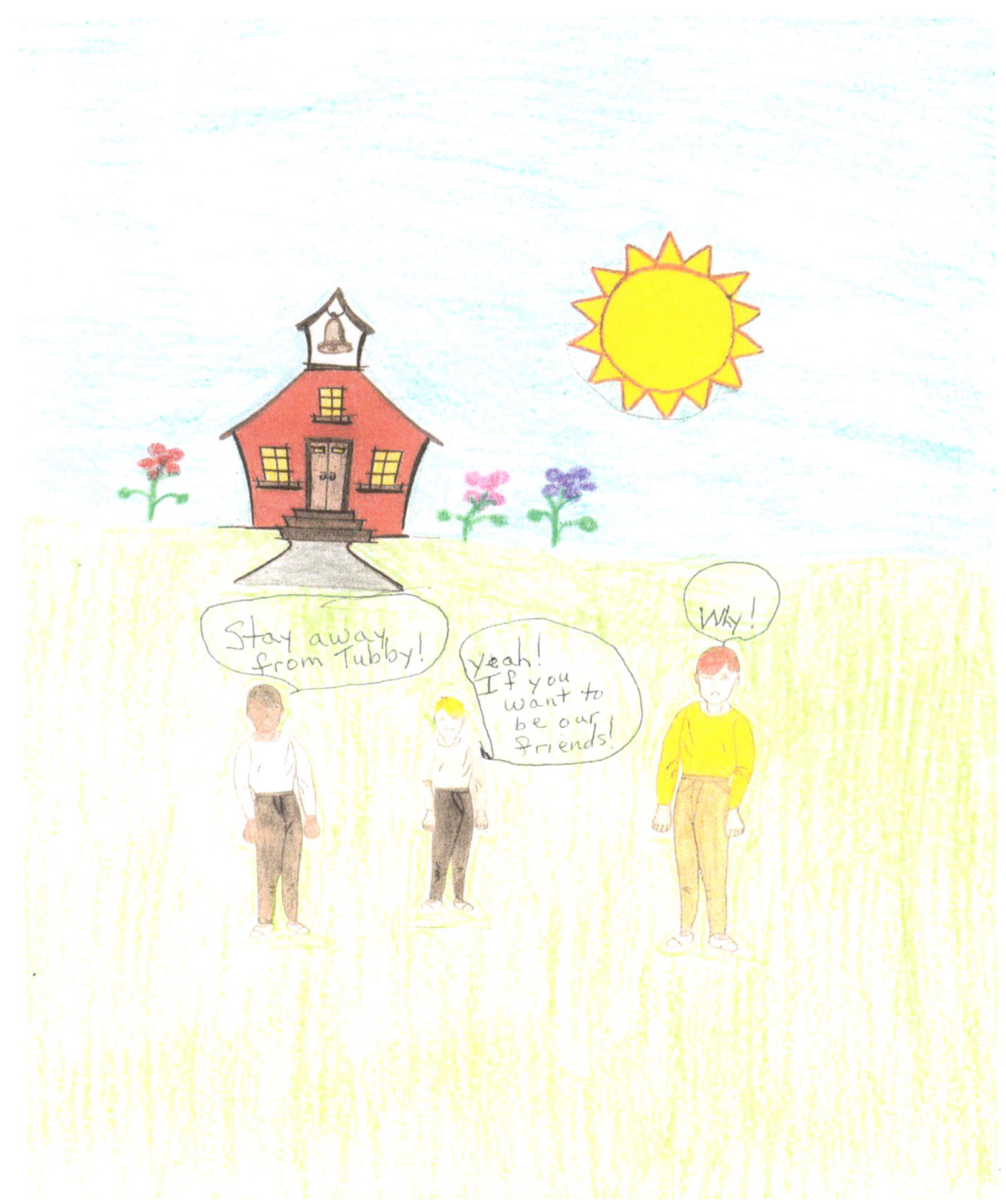

But, Mickey paid no attention to his friends and invited Tubby to his house to play.

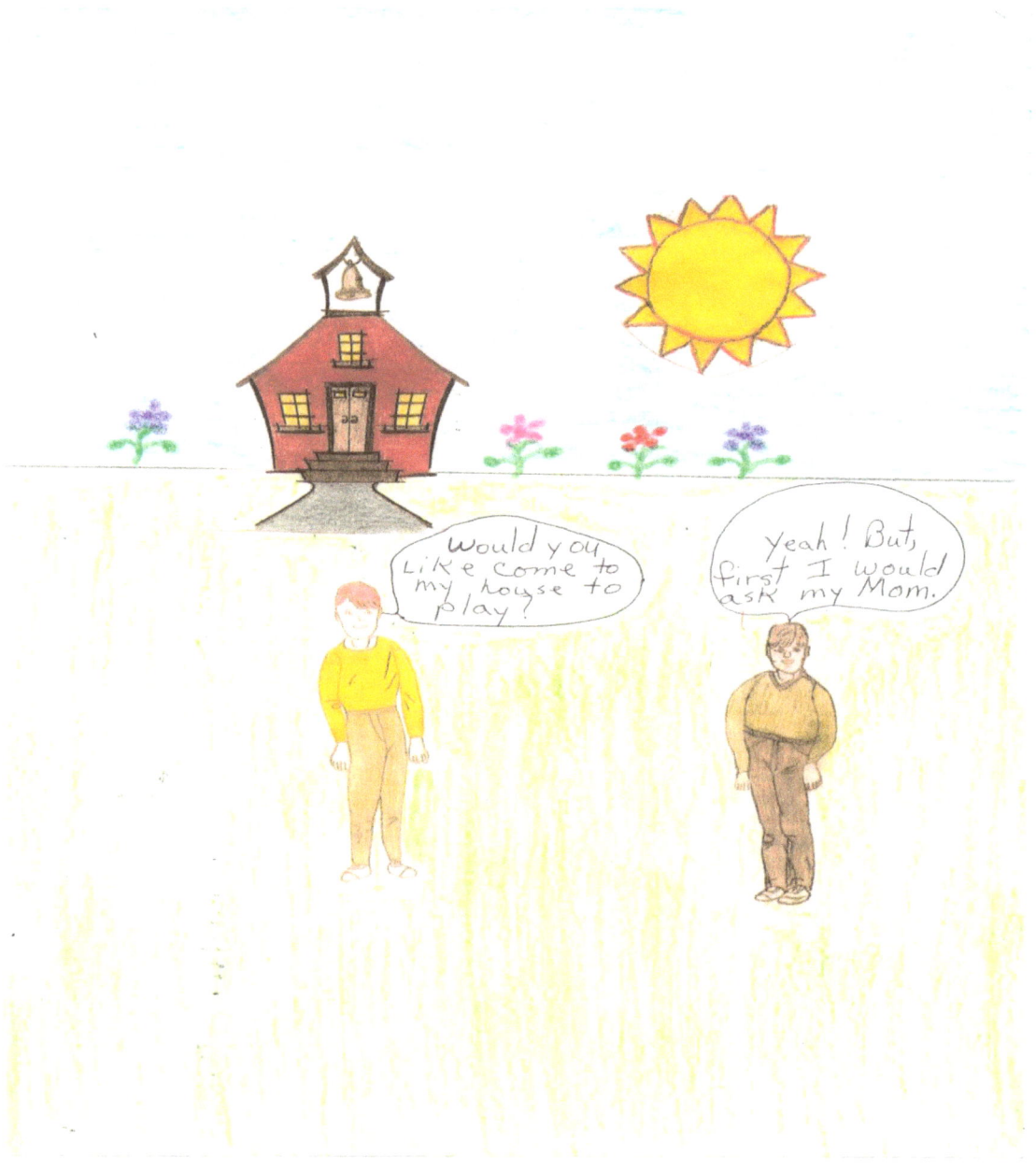

One day, Mickey and Sandy got together to find ways to help Fat Allie and Tubby to lose weight. What they decided to do is to take turns in using their homes for exercise and dancing for the four of them. But, the first thing to do is ask their mothers'. Mickey and Sandy's mothers said, "Yes." Sandy said to Mickey, "Let's go and let Allie and Tommy know that they can come to our homes to exercise and dance." Then, Mickey said, "Yeah!"

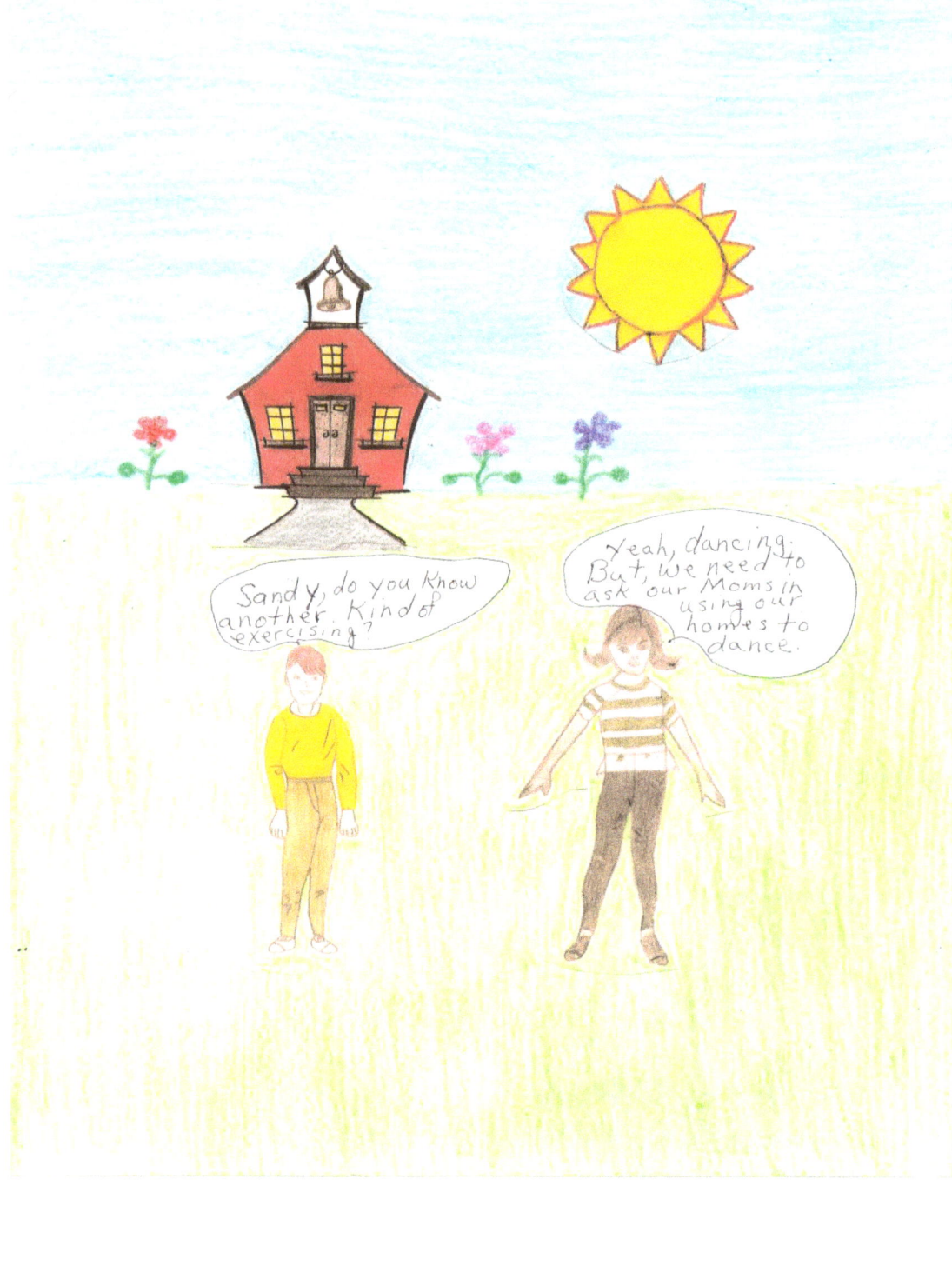

Both Sandy and Mickey invited Fat Allie and Tubby to do some exercise and dancing in their homes.

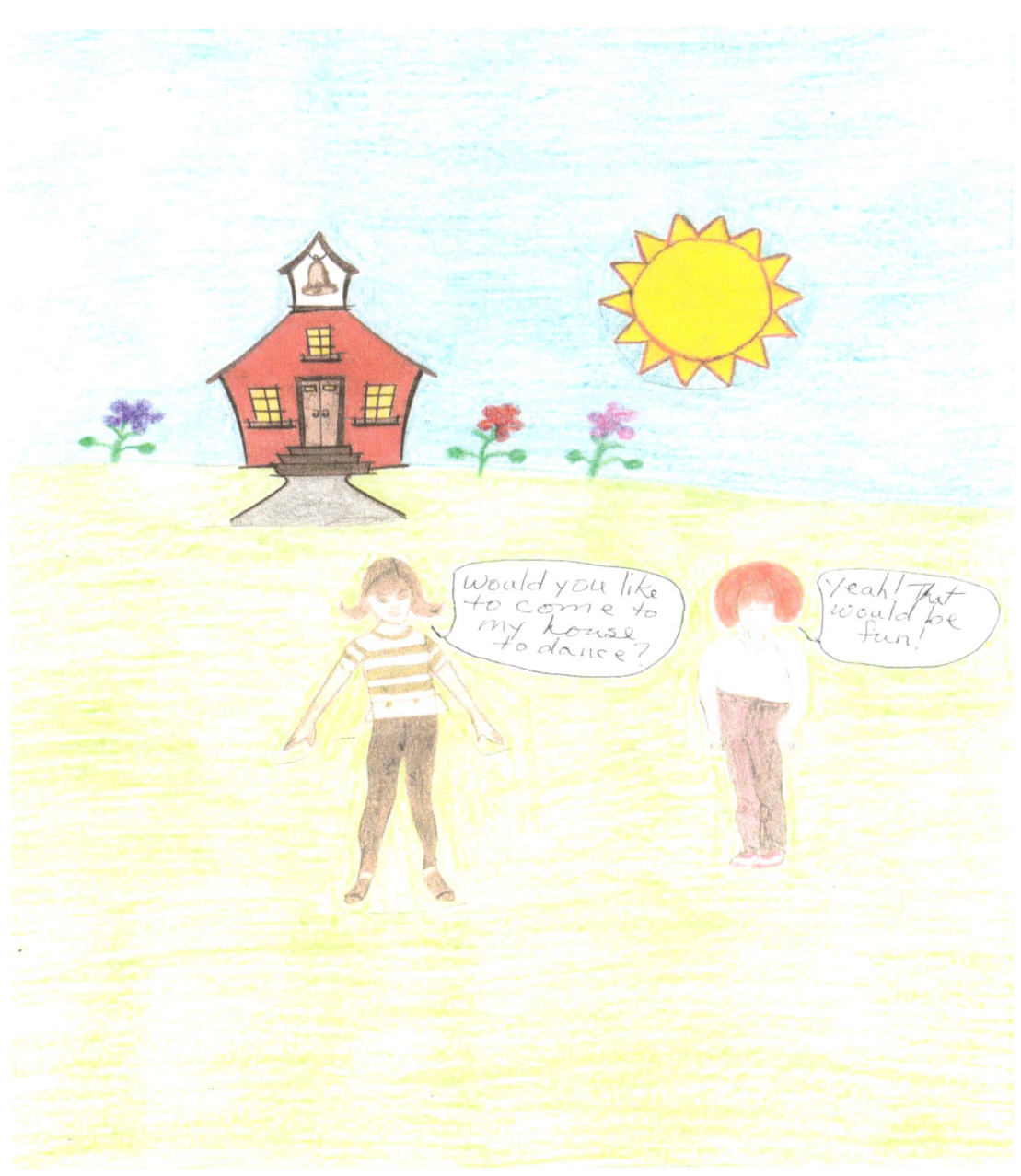

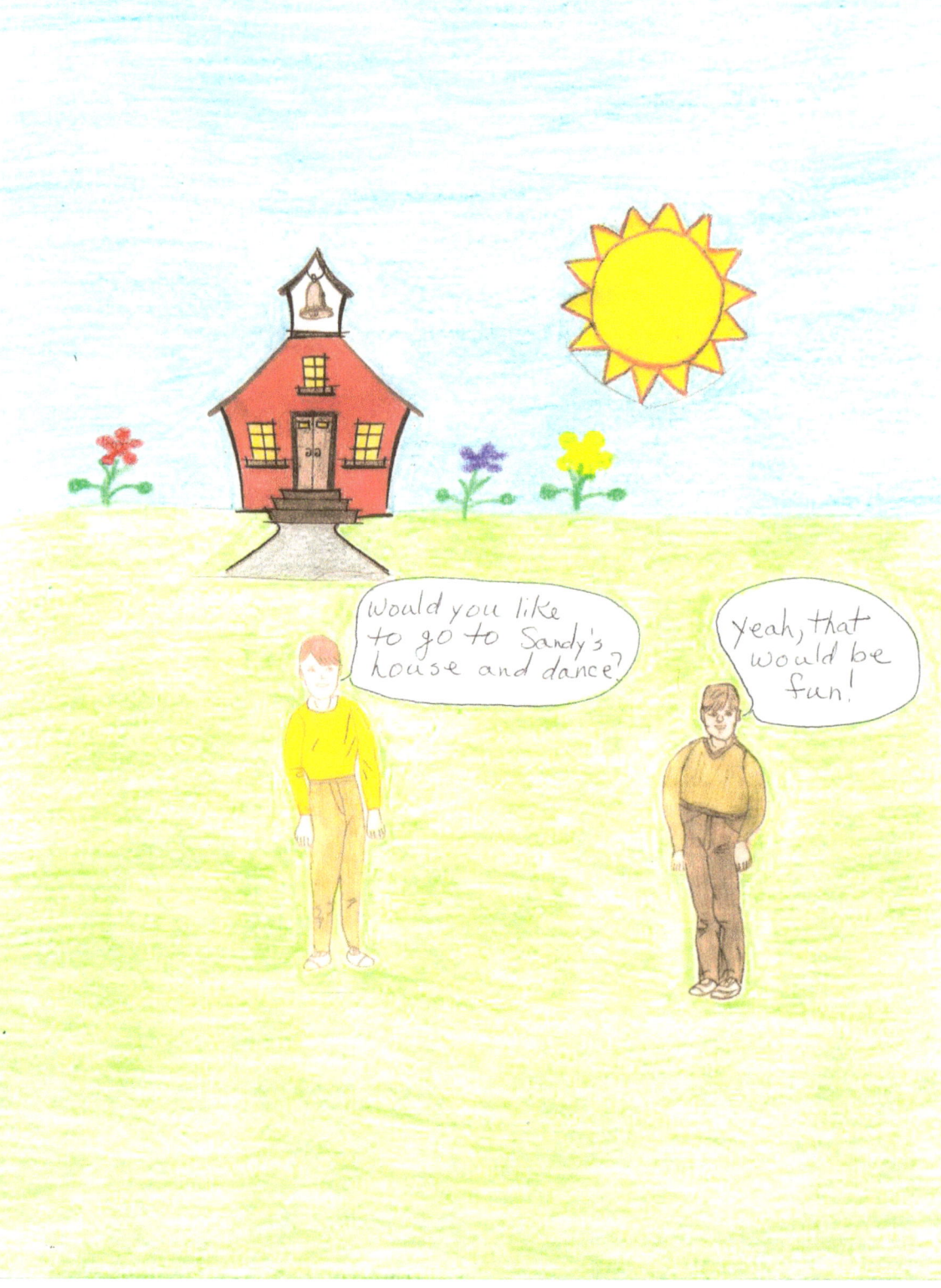

And, they all got together to do some exercise and dancing.

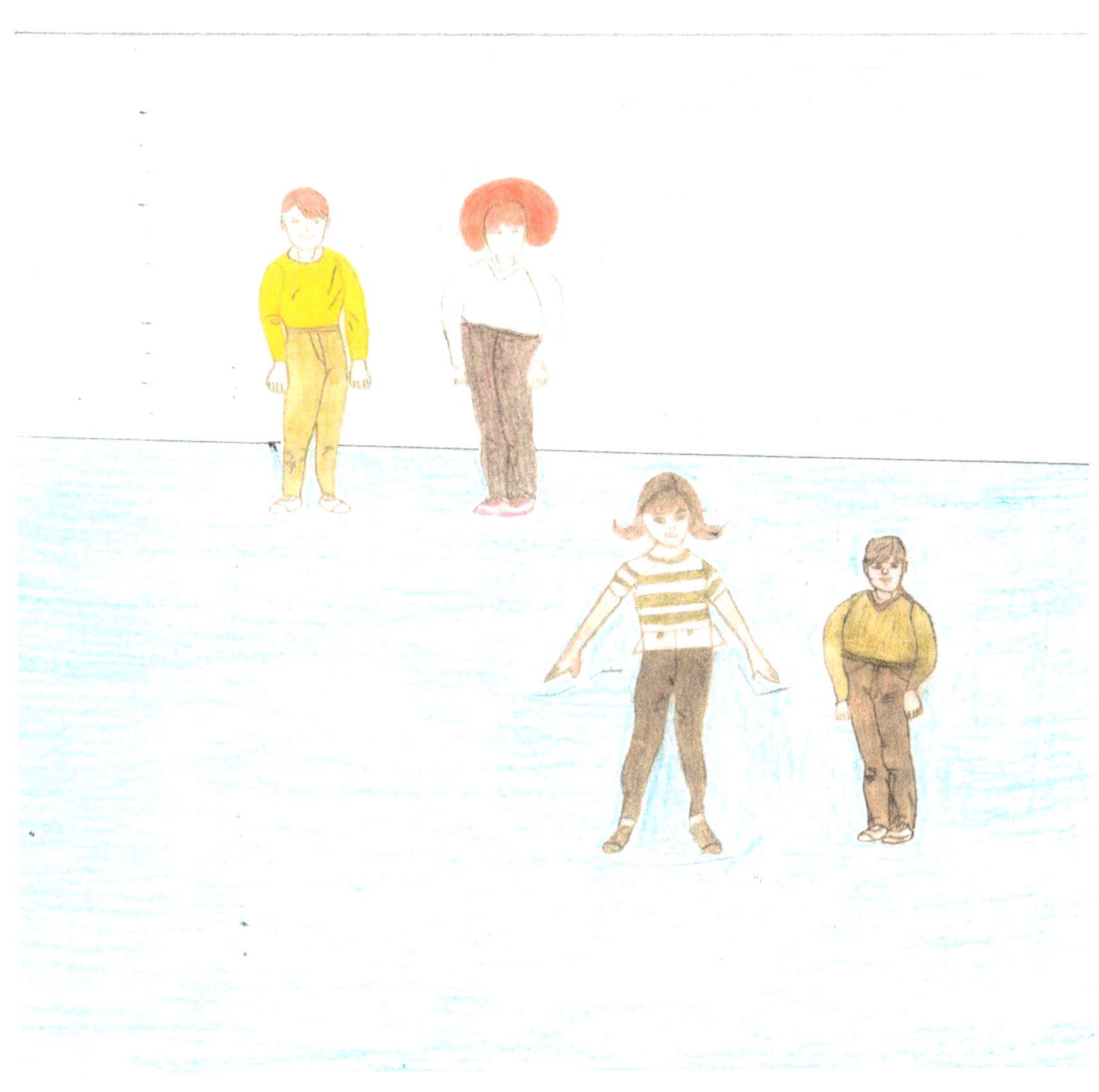

Sandy noticed that Fat Allie was eating the wrong kinds of food.

And Mickey found out that Tubby was eating the wrong kinds of food, too.

Sandy and Mickey noticed that Fat Allie and Tubby are not losing much

weight.

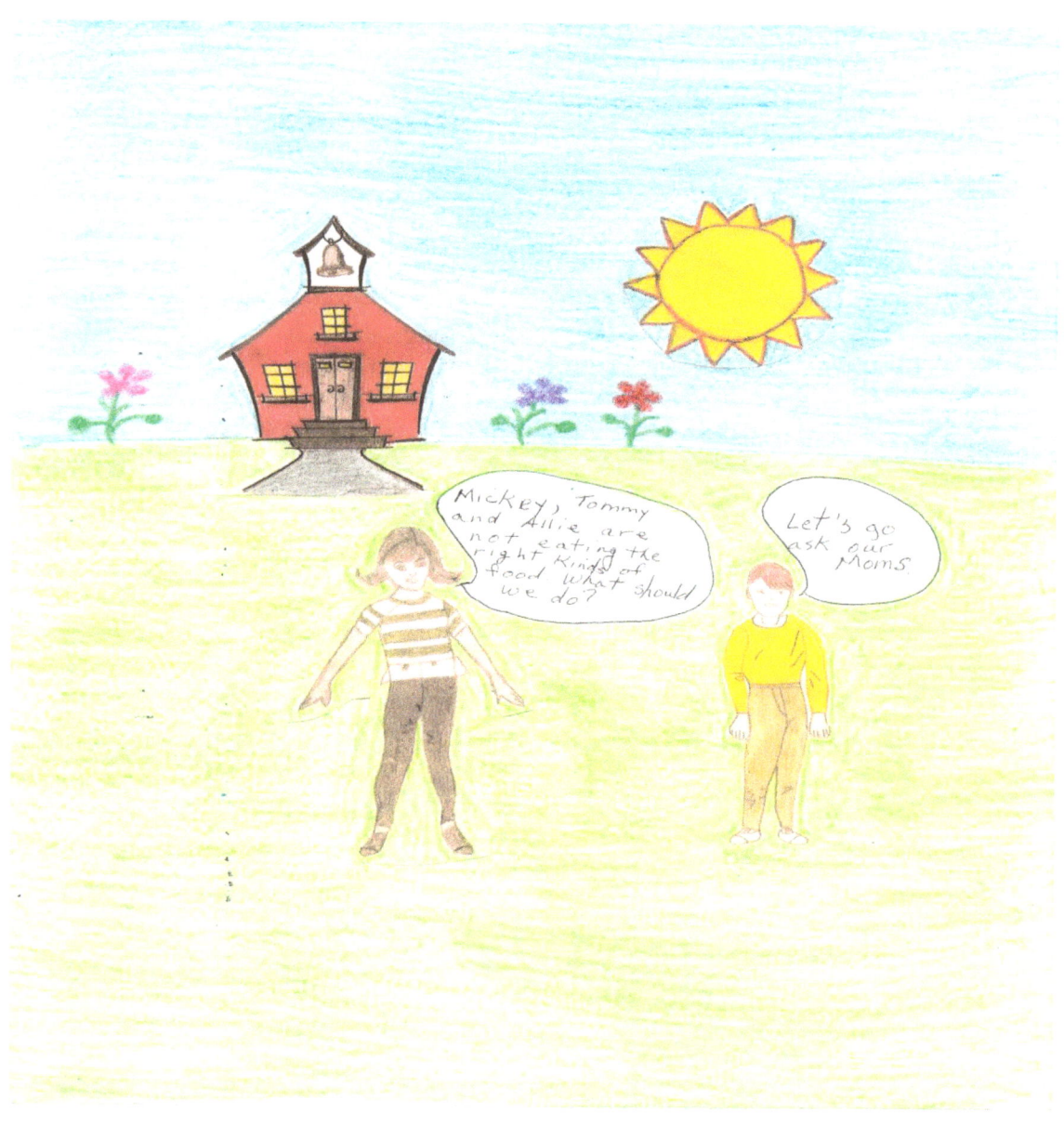

The mothers told them what healthy foods to eat for breakfast, lunch, dinner, and snacks.

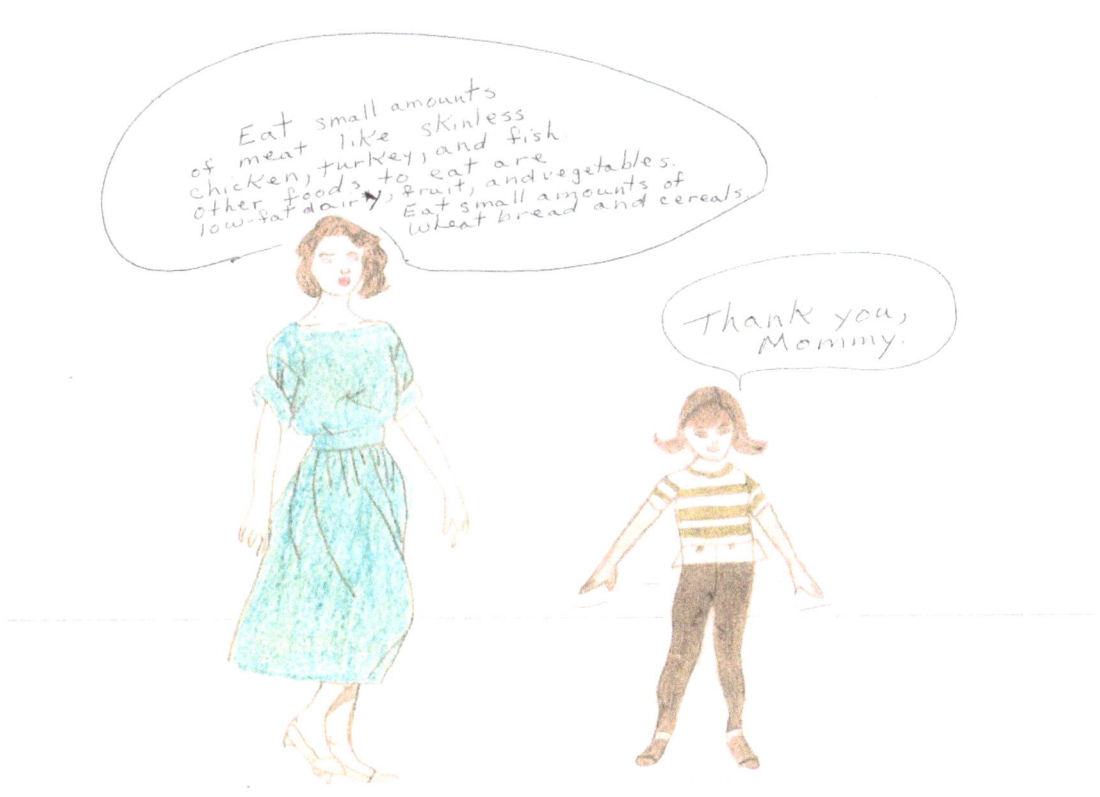

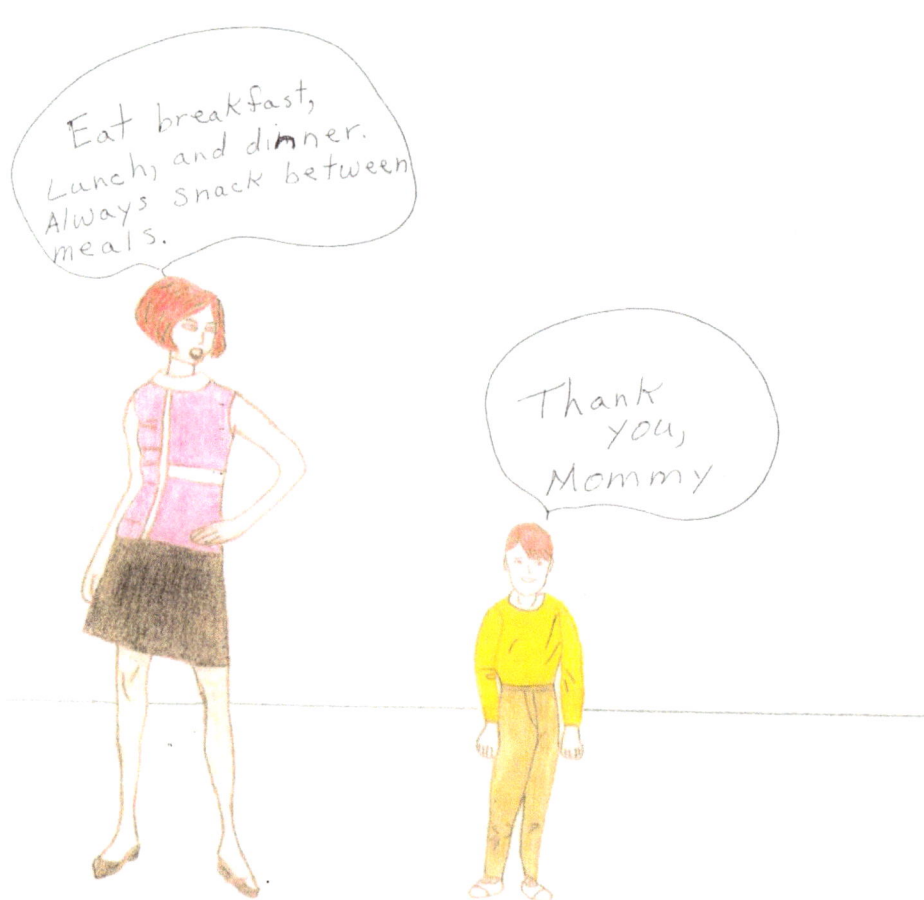

For Breakfast:

(1 each day)

1. Oatmeal with raisin and cinnamon along with fat-free milk

2. Two whole-wheat waffles with peanut butter and one banana

3. One egg, (scrambled, poached, or hard boiled) with vegetables along with one slice of whole-wheat toast with fruit jam.

4. One cup high fiber cereal with fruit and fat-free milk

For Lunch

(1 each day)

1. One peanut butter and jelly sandwich on whole-wheat bread with baby carrots

2. One tuna fish salad sandwich on whole-wheat bread with one slice low-fat cheese and baby spinach or romaine lettuce

3. One turkey sandwich on whole-wheat bread with one slice low-fat cheese and baby spinach or romaine lettuce

4. Egg salad sandwich on whole-wheat bread with slice low-fat cheese and baby spinach or romaine lettuce

For Dinner:

(1 each day)

1. One grilled turkey patty on whole-wheat roll along with vegetables

2. One grilled skinless barbecue chicken breast with Asian-style vegetables

3. One grilled fish with lemon juice along with peas and carrots

4. Small serving of brown rice with low-sodium chicken soup and vegetables

5. Small serving of sweet potatoes and lots of vegetables

6. Spinach and Romaine Salad with Strawberries and cooked cut-up chicken

Snacks:

(2 each day)

1. One slice low-fat cheese with an apple

2. One light non-fat yogurt with fruit

3. One slice whole-wheat bread with peanut butter and one banana

4. One 100 or fewer calorie snack

5. Two homemade low-fat whole-wheat cookies

6. One small pkg. raisins with one small pkg. of no salt nuts

7. Two scoops of low-fat or no-sugar ice cream

Make Your Own Meals:

1. Use small portions of wheat pasta like spaghetti with lots of vegetables or green beans

2. Eat small portions of meat with lots of vegetables

3. Make your own vegetable salads with low-fat meats (cooked)

Please Note:

Wheat pasta, brown rice, and sweet potatoes are starch that cannot be served with meat due to weight gain. Eat in moderation.

Two months later, Tubby and Fat Allie lost enough weight to look really good.

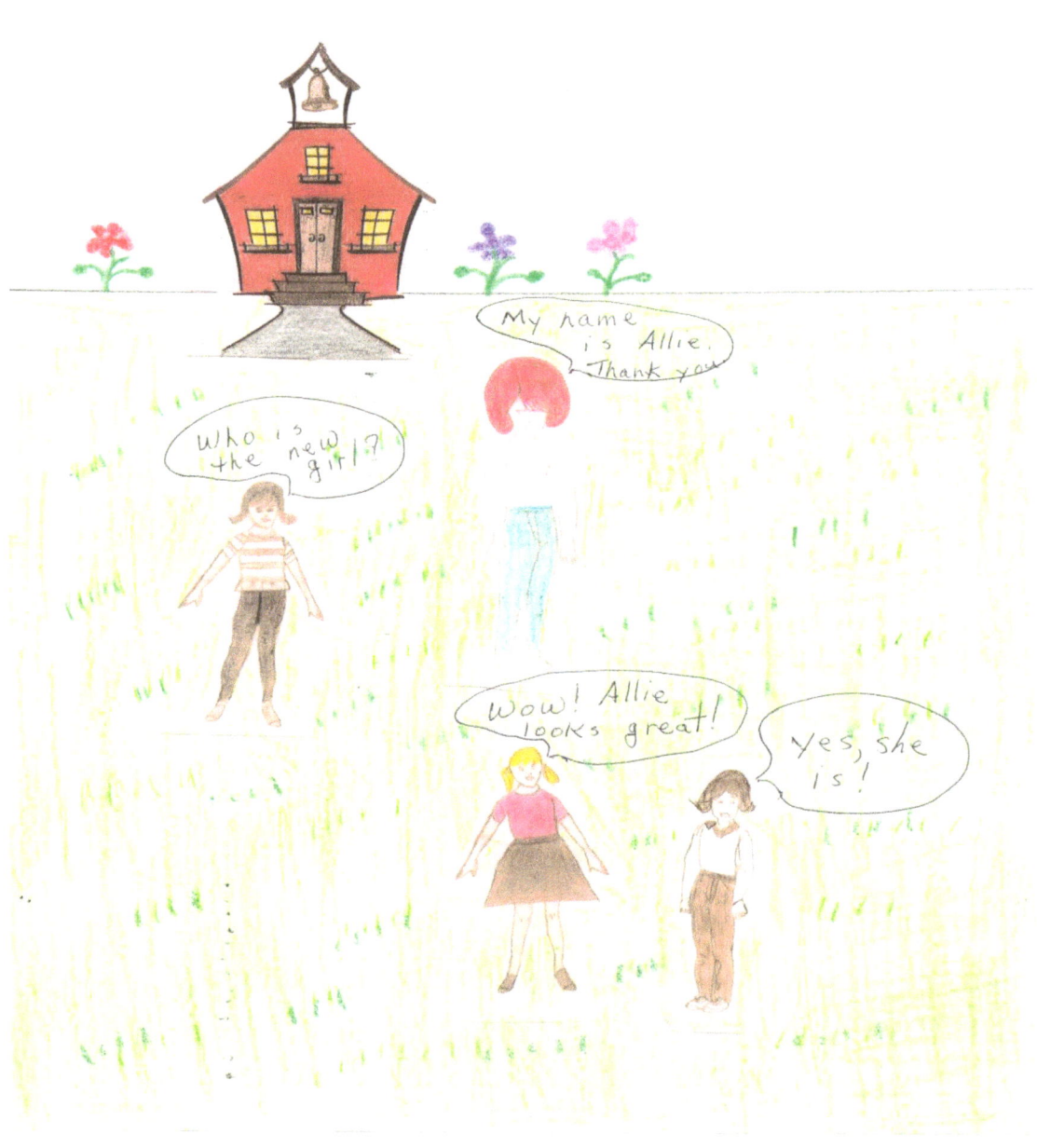

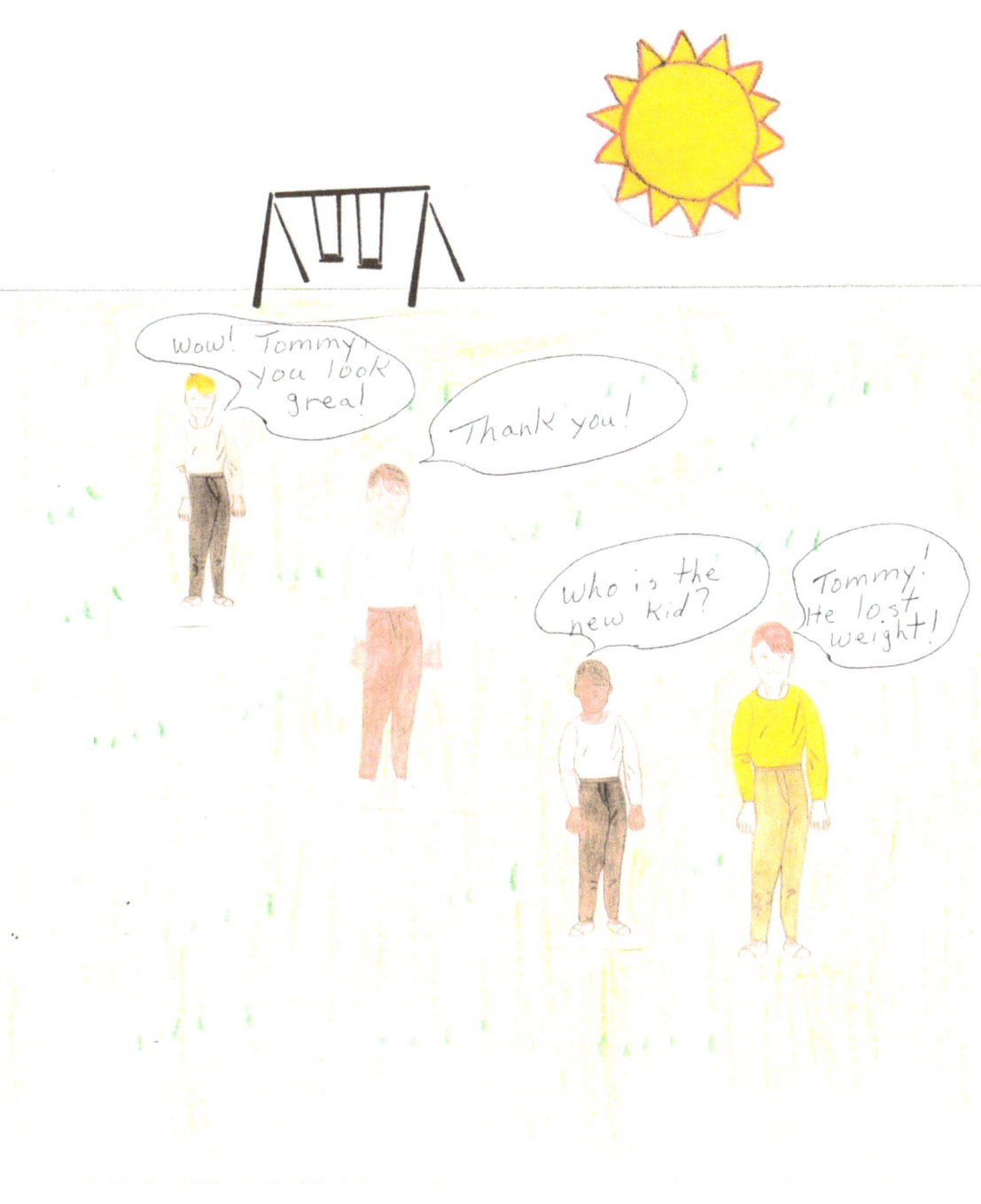

"Eating the right kinds of food and exercise will help us kids stay

healthy and strong."

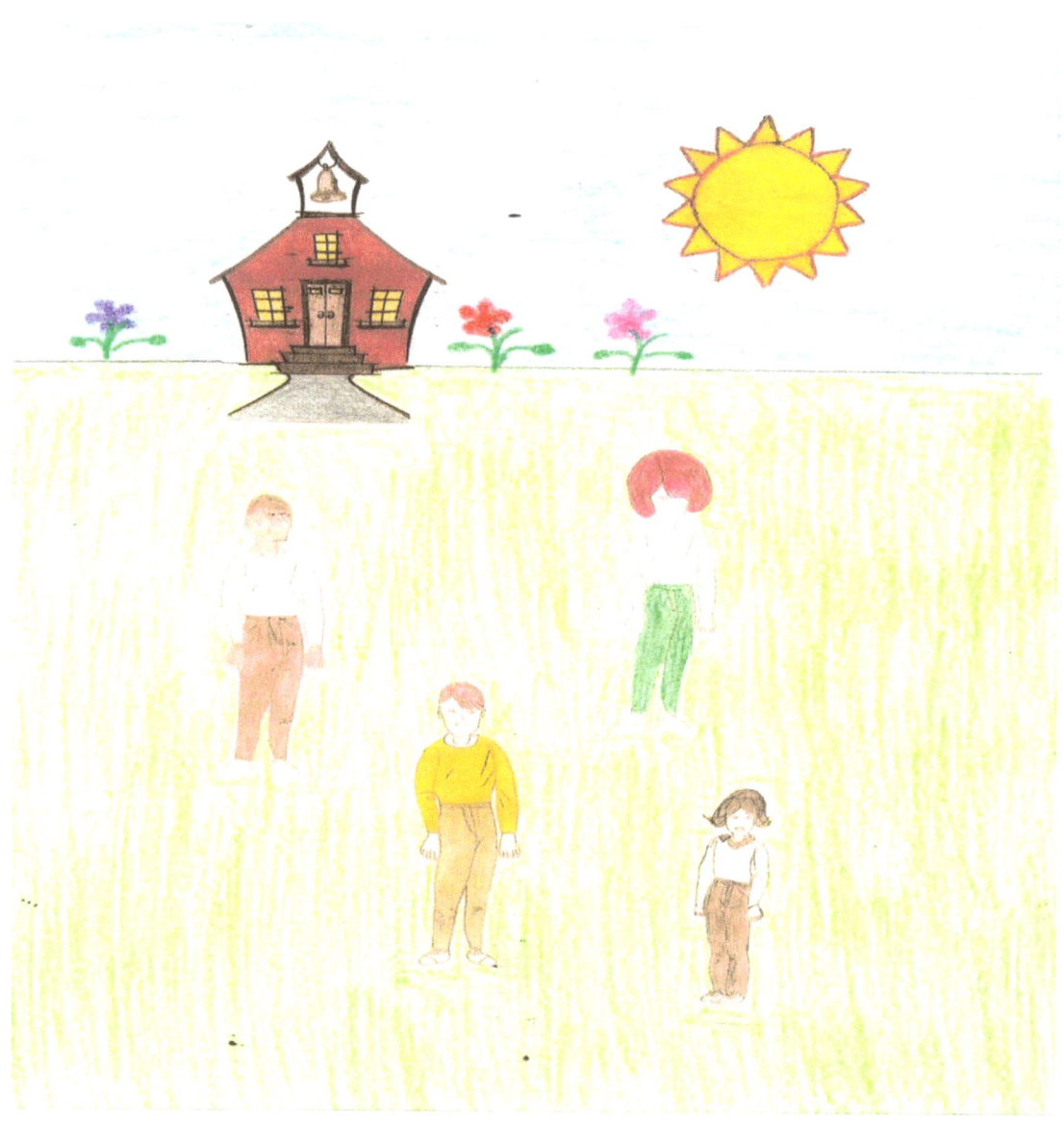

Tuna and Egg Salad

Ingredients:

4 eggs, hard-boiled

Romaine lettuce

2 cans light tuna w/water, drained

Pinch of ground ginger

Pinch of garlic powder

1 Tablespoon dried onions

Low-fat salad dressing

2 slices of whole-wheat bread

Peel eggs and cut small in bowl. With using fork, add tuna fish with ginger, garlic powder, and dried onions. Mix all ingredients together with salad dressing. By using fork, put ingredients on two slices of whole-wheat bread and add lettuce.

Turkey Meatloaf

Ingredients:

2 lbs. lean ground turkey

1 cup sweet onion or dried onion

½ tsp. garlic powder or minced garlic

2 egg whites

½ tsp. oregano

½ tsp. thyme

¼ cup ketchup

In large bowl, mix turkey, onion, garlic, egg whites, oregano, thyme, and ketchup. Put mixture in bread pan. Spread more ketchup on top of mixture. Bake 350 for 1 ¼ hours.

American Chop Suey

Ingredients:

1 lb. whole-wheat macaroni

1 jar of spaghetti sauce

1 (14.5 oz.) can stewed tomatoes

Cook macaroni for 7-8 minutes. Drain. Mix spaghetti sauce with stewed tomatoes in a large pan. Heat mixture and pour over macaroni. Serve with green beans.

Please note:

Add 1 lb. cooked turkey meat (optional)

Grilled Vegetables

Ingredients:

1 small zucchini

1 yellow pepper

1 sweet onion

¼ Tablespoon of butter

Preheat grill. Use three large aluminum foils for vegetables. Cut up zucchini, yellow pepper, and sweet onion and mix together. Pour mixture into foil and add butter. Cook on the grill for five minutes or until done. Place vegetables into a bowl. Serve hot or cold.

Broccoli with Cheese

Ingredients:

Minced garlic

2 lbs. broccoli florets

½ cup grated parmesan cheese or veg cheese

¼ Tablespoon butter

    Preheat grill. Mix together broccoli and minced garlic. Use three large aluminum foils and put broccoli mixed into the foil and add butter. Cover mixture and place on grill for five minutes or until done. Place broccoli mixture into bowl and mix parmesan cheese together. Serve hot.

Spinach Salad with Romaine Lettuce and Strawberries

Ingredients:

Spinach and Romaine Lettuce

1 package strawberries and 1 large apple

Celery, 1 cucumber, and 1 pepper

1sweet onion and 1 tomato

1 can crushed pineapple and 1 package cottage cheese

Raspberry Hazelnut Vinaigrette

Cut-up grilled chicken

Cut up all the ingredients and mix into large bowl. Add cottage cheese and Raspberry Hazelnut Vinaigrette into bowl and mix. Then, top with cut-up chicken.

Whole-Wheat Chocolate Chip Cookies

Ingredients:

1 cup margarine room temperature

1 cup brown sugar Splenda

1 teaspoon vanilla

2 eggs

2 cups whole wheat flour

1 teaspoon baking soda

1 teaspoon salt

1 package chocolate chips

Cream together margarine, sugar, and vanilla until light and fluffy. Add eggs and beat well. Combine flour, baking soda, and salt. Blend into mixture well. Stir in the chocolate chips. Drop teaspoonfuls, 2 inches apart on greased cookie sheet. Bake at 375 for 10-12 minutes. Makes about 8 dozen.

Please note:

Add ¾ cups chopped nuts (optional)